Mini Habits Weight Loss - Small Changes, Big Results

PUBLISHED by: Dorian Swift

Copyright © 2024. All right reserved.

Table of Contents

Introduction 4
Part 1: Understanding Mini Habits 16
    Chapter 1: The Concept of Mini Habits 16
    Chapter 2: The Psychology of Habit Formation 18
    Chapter 3: Why Traditional Diets Fail 20
    Chapter 4: Setting Realistic Goals 21
    Chapter 5: Creating Your Mini Habit Plan 23
Part 2: Mini Habits for Eating 27
    Chapter 6: Mindful Eating Techniques 27
    Chapter 7: Portion Control Strategies 29
    Chapter 8: Healthy Food Choices 31
    Chapter 9: Hydration Habits 34
    Chapter 10: Smart Snacking 35
    Chapter 11: Meal Planning and Preparation 37
    Chapter 12: Grocery Shopping Strategies 39
    Chapter 13: Overcoming Common Eating Challenges 40
Part 3: Mini Habits for Exercise 43
    Chapter 14: The Power of Daily Movement 43
    Chapter 15: Incorporating Strength Training 45
    Chapter 16: Making Cardio Fun 46
    Chapter 17: Flexibility and Stretching 48
    Chapter 18: Building an Exercise Routine 50
    Chapter 19: Overcoming Exercise Barriers 51

Chapter 20: Staying Active Throughout the Day 53

Part 4: Mindset and Motivation 55

Chapter 21: Understanding the Power of Mindset 55

Chapter 22: Setting SMART Goals 57

Chapter 23: Building a Support System 59

Chapter 24: Overcoming Plateaus 60

Chapter 25: Dealing with Setbacks 62

Chapter 26: Cultivating Patience and Persistence 64

Chapter 27: Creating a Positive Environment 65

Chapter 28: Practicing Mindfulness and Stress Management 67

Chapter 29: Building Self-Discipline 68

Chapter 30: Embracing the Journey 70

Conclusion: The Journey to Lasting Weight Loss 73

10 Motivational Quotes for Weight Loss 83

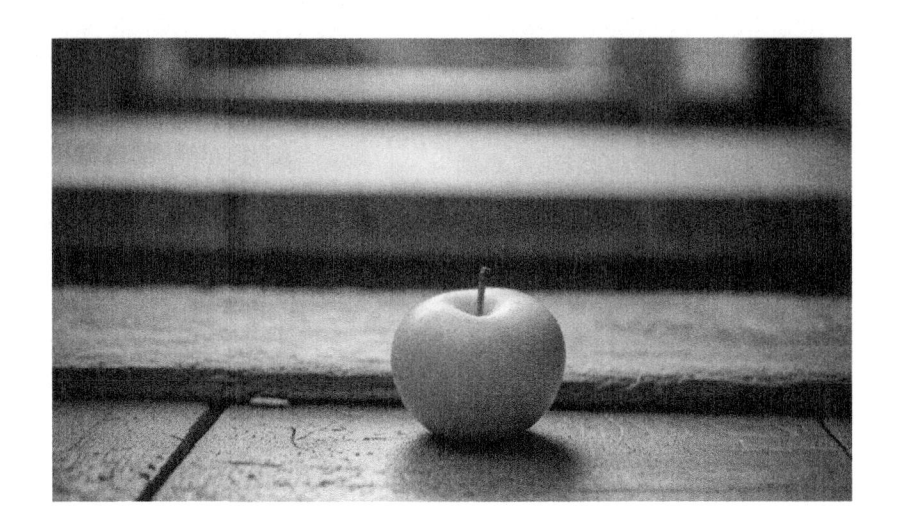

Introduction

Small steps every day

The Power of Mini Habits for Weight Loss

Welcome to "Mini Habits for Weight Loss: Small Changes, Big Results." This book is designed to help you transform your approach to weight loss through the implementation of small, manageable habits. In this introduction, we will explore the concept of mini habits, the science behind why they work, and how you can start incorporating them into your daily life for lasting weight loss and a healthier lifestyle.

Understanding Mini Habits

Mini habits are tiny, almost ridiculously small behaviors that are easy to incorporate into your daily routine. Unlike traditional goals that often require significant effort and can lead to burnout, mini habits are so small that they are virtually impossible to fail. The idea is to lower the barrier to action so much that you can't help but succeed.

For example, instead of setting a goal to exercise for an hour every day, you might start with a mini habit of doing one push-up per day. This tiny commitment is easy to accomplish and, importantly, it builds momentum. Once you've done one push-up, you're more likely to do more. This concept can be applied to various aspects of weight loss, from dietary changes to physical activity, and even to mental and emotional well-being.

The Problem with Traditional Diets

Traditional diets and weight loss programs often promise quick results through drastic changes. While these methods can work in the short term, they are usually unsustainable. People often revert to their old habits once the initial motivation wears off, leading to a cycle of weight loss and gain. This cycle, known as yo-yo dieting, can be damaging both physically and mentally.

The problem with these conventional approaches is that they require a significant amount of willpower and motivation, which are finite resources. When you rely solely on willpower to make large changes, you are setting yourself up for failure. Life's challenges, stress, and fatigue can easily derail your efforts, leaving you feeling discouraged and defeated.

Why Mini Habits Work

The power of mini habits lies in their simplicity and consistency. Here's why they are so effective:

Reduced Resistance: Mini habits are so small that they do not trigger resistance. For example, if your mini habit is to drink one glass of water first thing in the morning, it's a simple task that doesn't require much effort or motivation.

Consistency Over Intensity: By focusing on small, consistent actions, you build a solid foundation for lasting change. Consistency is key to forming new habits, and mini habits make it easier to maintain that consistency.

Momentum and Motivation: Completing a mini habit gives you a sense of accomplishment, which can boost your motivation to do more. This creates a positive feedback loop where small successes lead to bigger ones.

Positive Reinforcement: Because mini habits are easy to achieve, they provide frequent positive reinforcement. This reinforces the behavior and makes it more likely to become a lasting habit.

Building Confidence: Successfully completing mini habits builds your confidence. As you accumulate small wins, you start to believe in your ability to make changes, which can lead to tackling bigger challenges.

Setting the Foundation for Mini Habits

Before you start implementing mini habits for weight loss, it's important to set a solid foundation. This involves understanding your goals, breaking them down into manageable mini habits, and creating a plan to integrate them into your daily routine.

Identifying Your Goals

The first step is to clearly define your weight loss goals. It's important to be specific and realistic. Instead of a vague goal like "lose weight," set a specific target such as "lose 10 pounds in three months." Once you have a clear goal, you can break it down into smaller, actionable steps.

Breaking Down Goals into Mini Habits

Next, take your larger goal and break it down into mini habits. For instance, if your goal is to lose 10 pounds, you might start with mini habits like:

- Drinking a glass of water before each meal.
- Walking for five minutes after lunch.
- Adding one serving of vegetables to your dinner.

These mini habits are small enough to be manageable but are also aligned with your larger goal. As you consistently practice these mini habits, they will accumulate and contribute to your weight loss.

Creating a Mini Habit Plan

Once you've identified your mini habits, create a plan to integrate them into your daily routine. Choose a specific time or trigger for each habit. For example, you might decide to drink a glass of water as soon as you wake up or walk for five minutes right after lunch. The key is to make the habit easy to remember and incorporate into your existing routine.

Building Your Mini Habits

Now that you have a plan, it's time to start building your mini habits. Here are some tips to help you get started and stay on track:

Start Small and Be Consistent

Remember, the goal is to make the habit so small that it's almost impossible to fail. Start with the tiniest version of the habit and focus on consistency. It's better to do a small habit every day than to aim for a larger habit that you can't sustain.

Track Your Progress

Keep track of your mini habits to monitor your progress and stay motivated. You can use a habit tracker, a journal, or a simple checklist. Seeing your progress can provide a sense of accomplishment and motivate you to keep going.

Celebrate Small Wins

Celebrate your successes, no matter how small. Acknowledge and reward yourself for completing your mini habits. This positive reinforcement can help reinforce the behavior and make it more likely to stick.

Adjust and Adapt

As you progress, you may need to adjust your mini habits. If a habit becomes too easy, you can gradually increase its intensity. For example, if you started with one push-up per day, you might increase it to two or three. The key is to make small, incremental changes that build on your success.

Mini Habits for Eating

One of the most effective ways to achieve weight loss is through mindful eating. Mini habits can help you develop a healthier relationship with food and make better choices without feeling deprived.

Mindful Eating

Mindful eating involves paying full attention to the experience of eating. It's about savoring each bite and being aware of hunger and fullness cues. Mini habits for mindful eating might include:

- Taking a few deep breaths before starting your meal.
- Putting your fork down between bites.
- Chewing each bite thoroughly.

Portion Control

Controlling portion sizes is crucial for weight loss. Mini habits can help you manage portions without feeling like you're missing out. Examples of mini habits for portion control include:

- Using smaller plates and bowls.
- Serving yourself smaller portions and going back for seconds only if you're still hungry.
- Avoiding eating directly from the package.

Healthy Food Choices

Making healthier food choices can have a significant impact on your weight loss journey. Mini habits for healthier eating might include:

- Adding one serving of vegetables to your meals.
- Swapping sugary snacks for fruit.
- Choosing whole grains instead of refined grains.

Mini Habits for Exercise

Physical activity is an essential component of weight loss and overall health. Mini habits can help you incorporate more movement into your day without feeling overwhelmed.

Starting Small

If you're new to exercise or have been inactive for a while, start with very small, manageable activities. Mini habits for starting an exercise routine might include:

- Doing one push-up or squat each day.
- Taking a five-minute walk during your lunch break.
- Stretching for a few minutes before bed.

Building Consistency

The key to successful exercise is consistency. Mini habits can help you build a regular exercise routine. Examples include:

- Scheduling a specific time each day for a short workout.
- Setting a reminder to stand up and move every hour.
- Joining a fitness class or finding a workout buddy for accountability.

Increasing Intensity Gradually

As you build consistency, you can gradually increase the intensity of your workouts. Mini habits for increasing intensity might include:

- Adding one extra minute to your daily walk each week.
- Increasing the number of repetitions in your strength training exercises.
- Trying a new form of exercise, such as yoga or cycling.

Lifestyle and Mindset

Achieving and maintaining weight loss involves more than just diet and exercise. It also requires a healthy lifestyle and a positive mindset. Mini habits can help you manage stress, improve sleep, and build a supportive environment.

Managing Stress

Stress can have a significant impact on weight loss. Mini habits for stress management might include:

- Practicing deep breathing exercises for a few minutes each day.
- Taking short breaks to relax and unwind.
- Engaging in a hobby or activity that you enjoy.

Improving Sleep

Sleep plays a crucial role in weight management. Mini habits for better sleep might include:

- Establishing a regular bedtime routine.
- Limiting screen time before bed.

Creating a comfortable sleep environment.

Building a Supportive Environment

Surrounding yourself with a supportive environment can make a big difference in your weight loss journey. Mini habits for building a supportive environment might include:

- Sharing your goals with a friend or family member.
- Joining a support group or online community.
- Keeping healthy snacks and meals readily available.

Tracking Progress and Staying Motivated

Monitoring your progress and celebrating your successes can help you stay motivated. Mini habits for tracking progress might include:

- Keeping a daily journal of your mini habits and achievements.
- Setting small, achievable milestones and rewarding yourself when you reach them.
- Reflecting on your progress regularly and adjusting your mini habits as needed.
-

Embracing the Journey

Weight loss is a journey, not a destination. By focusing on mini habits, you can make sustainable changes that lead to lasting results. Remember to be patient with yourself and embrace the process. Celebrate your small wins and learn from any setbacks.

In this book, you'll find practical, actionable steps to help you implement mini habits for weight loss. Each chapter will provide detailed guidance on specific habits, along with tips for overcoming challenges and staying motivated. By the end of this book, you'll have a comprehensive plan to achieve your weight loss goals through small, consistent actions.

Thank you for embarking on this journey with me. I'm excited to help you transform your approach to weight loss and discover the power of mini habits. Let's get started!

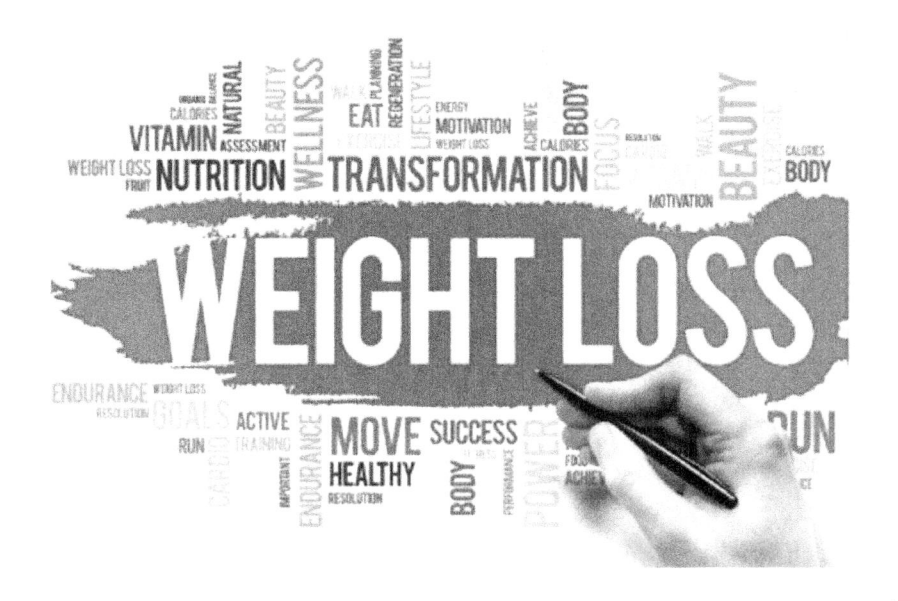

Part 1: Understanding Mini Habits

Chapter 1: The Concept of Mini Habits

> *"Just believe in yourself.*
> *Even if you don't, pretend that you do,*
> *and at some point, you will."*
> Venus Williams

What Are Mini Habits?

Mini habits are small, easy-to-accomplish actions that can be integrated into your daily routine with minimal effort. The idea is to start so small that it's almost impossible to fail. For example, instead of committing to a 30-minute workout every day, you start with one push-up or a 5-

minute walk. These mini habits require little motivation, making them easier to stick to and gradually build upon.

The Origin of Mini Habits

The concept of mini habits was popularized by Stephen Guise in his book, Mini Habits: Smaller Habits, Bigger Results. Guise discovered that by lowering the bar for success, he was able to build consistent behaviors that led to significant improvements in his life. This approach is grounded in behavioral psychology, emphasizing the power of small, incremental changes over time.

Benefits of Mini Habits

- Reduced Resistance: Mini habits are so small that they don't trigger significant resistance or procrastination.
- Easy to Start: Because they require minimal effort, starting a mini habit is easy, which is often the biggest hurdle.
- Consistency: Mini habits promote consistency, which is crucial for long-term success.
- Flexibility: They can be adapted to fit any lifestyle or schedule.
- Cumulative Effect: Over time, small actions add up to substantial changes and improvements.

Examples of Mini Habits

- Drinking one glass of water before each meal.
- Doing one push-up every day.
- Walking for five minutes after lunch.
- Adding one serving of vegetables to your dinner.
- Meditating for one minute before bed.

By starting with these tiny actions, you create a foundation for more significant changes. The key is to make the habit so small that you can't say no.

Chapter 2: The Psychology of Habit Formation

Understanding the Habit Loop

Habits are formed through a three-step loop: cue, routine, and reward. This loop is ingrained in our brains, making habitual behaviors automatic and consistent.

- **Cue:** This is the trigger that initiates the habit. It can be a time of day, an emotional state, or an action.
- **Routine:** This is the behavior or action you want to turn into a habit.
- **Reward:** This is the benefit you get from the behavior, which reinforces the habit.

By understanding this loop, you can create new habits by establishing clear cues and rewarding yourself for following through.

The Power of Small Wins

Small wins are achievements that might seem insignificant on their own but collectively lead to big changes. Each small win boosts your confidence and motivation, making it easier to achieve the next small win. This creates a positive feedback loop, reinforcing the habit and encouraging continuous improvement.

Overcoming Willpower Depletion

Willpower is a finite resource. When you rely on willpower alone to make significant changes, you're likely to experience fatigue and burnout. Mini habits bypass this issue by requiring minimal effort and willpower. They help you build a habit with little resistance, preserving your willpower for more challenging tasks.

The Role of Consistency

Consistency is critical for habit formation. It's better to perform a small habit daily than to do something significant sporadically. Consistent actions reinforce the habit loop, making the behavior automatic over time. Mini habits ensure that you maintain this consistency by setting achievable daily goals.

Chapter 3: Why Traditional Diets Fail

The Pitfalls of Traditional Diets

Traditional diets often involve drastic changes and strict rules. While they can lead to quick weight loss, they are usually unsustainable for several reasons:

- **High Expectations:** Drastic changes require a lot of effort and willpower, which can be overwhelming.
- **Deprivation:** Restrictive diets can lead to feelings of deprivation and resentment, increasing the likelihood of binge eating.
- **Short-Term Focus:** Many diets are designed for rapid weight loss rather than long-term maintenance.
- **Lack of Flexibility:** Strict rules don't account for the complexities of everyday life, making them hard to stick to.

The Cycle of Yo-Yo Dieting

Yo-yo dieting refers to the cycle of losing weight, regaining it, and then dieting again. This cycle is harmful to both physical and mental health. It often results from diets that are too restrictive, causing individuals to revert to old eating habits once the diet ends. This pattern can lead to feelings of failure and frustration.

Sustainability vs. Quick Fixes

Sustainable weight loss requires changes that can be maintained over the long term. Quick fixes might provide immediate results, but they don't address the underlying habits that led to weight gain. Mini habits offer a sustainable approach by focusing on small, manageable changes that can be easily maintained.

The Benefits of a Habit-Based Approach

A habit-based approach to weight loss focuses on creating lasting changes in behavior rather than short-term fixes. By building healthy habits gradually, you can achieve long-term weight loss and a healthier lifestyle. Mini habits make this process manageable and effective, ensuring that you develop habits that stick.

Chapter 4: Setting Realistic Goals

The Importance of Realistic Goals

Setting realistic goals is crucial for success. Unrealistic goals can lead to disappointment and frustration, while realistic goals provide a clear and achievable path forward. When goals are attainable, they motivate you to keep going and build confidence in your ability to succeed.

SMART Goals

SMART is an acronym for Specific, Measurable, Achievable, Relevant, and Time-bound. Setting SMART goals ensures that your objectives are clear and attainable.

- **Specific:** Clearly define what you want to achieve.
- **Measurable:** Ensure that you can track your progress.
- **Achievable:** Set goals that are realistic and attainable.
- **Relevant:** Choose goals that are meaningful and aligned with your overall objectives.
- **Time-bound:** Set a deadline for achieving your goals.

Breaking Down Big Goals into Mini Habits

Once you've set your goals, break them down into smaller, manageable mini habits. For example, if your goal is to lose 20 pounds in six months, your mini habits might include:

- Drinking a glass of water before meals.
- Eating a serving of vegetables with every meal.

Walking for 10 minutes every day.

These mini habits are directly aligned with your larger goal and are easy to implement on a daily basis.

Tracking Your Progress

Tracking your progress is essential for staying motivated and making adjustments as needed. Use a journal, app, or habit tracker to record your daily mini habits and monitor your progress. Seeing your progress over time can provide a sense of accomplishment and encourage you to keep going.

Celebrating Small Wins

Celebrate your successes, no matter how small. Recognize and reward yourself for completing your mini habits and achieving milestones. This positive reinforcement can boost your motivation and reinforce the behavior, making it more likely to stick.

Chapter 5: Creating Your Mini Habit Plan

Designing a Personalized Mini Habit Plan

Creating a personalized mini habit plan involves identifying the habits that will help you achieve your goals and integrating them into your daily routine. Follow these steps to design your plan:

- **Identify Your Goals:** Clearly define your weight loss goals using the SMART criteria.
- **Break Down Goals into Mini Habits:** Identify the small, manageable actions that will help you achieve your goals.
- **Choose Specific Times or Triggers:** Decide when and how you will perform each mini habit. Link them

to existing routines or specific triggers to make them easier to remember.
- **Start Small:** Begin with the smallest version of the habit to ensure success.
- **Track Your Progress:** Use a journal, app, or habit tracker to monitor your daily habits and progress.
- **Adjust as Needed:** Be flexible and adjust your habits as needed. If a habit becomes too easy, gradually increase its intensity.

Integrating Mini Habits into Your Daily Routine

Integrate your mini habits into your existing routine to make them easier to remember and perform. For example:

- Morning Routine: Drink a glass of water as soon as you wake up.
- Work Routine: Take a five-minute walk during your lunch break.
- Evening Routine: Add a serving of vegetables to your dinner.

By linking mini habits to existing routines, you create a seamless transition and reduce the likelihood of forgetting or skipping the habit.

Overcoming Common Challenges

Implementing new habits can come with challenges. Here are some common obstacles and how to overcome them:

Forgetting: Use reminders, alarms, or habit tracking apps to help you remember your mini habits.

- **Lack of Motivation:** Start with the smallest possible habit to ensure success and build momentum.
- **Time Constraints:** Choose mini habits that require minimal time and can be easily integrated into your routine.
- **Setbacks:** Expect setbacks and don't be discouraged by them. Reflect on what caused the setback and adjust your plan as needed.

Maintaining Flexibility

Flexibility is key to long-term success. Life is unpredictable, and there will be days when it's challenging to stick to your habits. Allow yourself some grace and be willing to adapt your plan as needed. The goal is to maintain consistency over time, not perfection.

The Long-Term Perspective

Remember that weight loss and habit formation are long-term endeavors. Focus on making small, sustainable changes that you can maintain over time. By building a solid foundation of mini habits, you create a path to lasting weight loss and a healthier lifestyle.

Conclusion of Part 1

Understanding the power of mini habits is the first step towards achieving your weight loss goals. By starting small, focusing on consistency, and creating a personalized mini habit plan, you set yourself up for long-term success. In the following sections, we will delve deeper into specific mini habits for eating, exercise, and lifestyle changes, providing you with practical tools and strategies to continue your journey towards a healthier you.

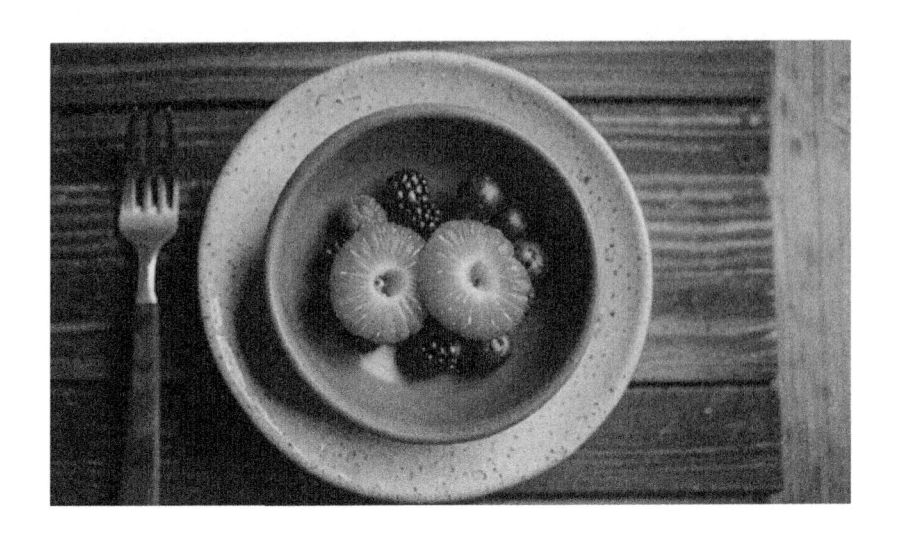

Part 2: Mini Habits for Eating

"Every accomplishment starts with a decision to try."

Chapter 6: Mindful Eating Techniques

Understanding Mindful Eating

Mindful eating is a practice that encourages full awareness of the eating experience, including sensations, emotions, and behaviors associated with food. By practicing mindfulness during meals, individuals can develop a healthier relationship with food and make more conscious choices.

Mini Habits for Mindful Eating

Savor Each Bite: Take the time to fully experience the flavors, textures, and aromas of your food. Chew slowly and mindfully, paying attention to how each bite feels in your mouth.

Eat Without Distractions: Avoid eating in front of the TV, computer, or smartphone. Instead, focus solely on the act of eating and the sensory experience it provides.

Listen to Your Body: Tune in to your body's hunger and fullness signals. Eat when you're hungry and stop when you're satisfied, even if there's food left on your plate.

Practice Gratitude: Before starting your meal, take a moment to express gratitude for the food in front of you. This can help cultivate a positive mindset and appreciation for the nourishment your body receives.

Pause Between Bites: Put your fork down between bites and take a moment to check in with yourself. Assess your hunger levels and ask yourself if you're truly enjoying the food.

Benefits of Mindful Eating

- **Improved Digestion:** Mindful eating promotes thorough chewing and digestion, leading to better nutrient absorption and reduced digestive discomfort.
- **Weight Management:** By paying attention to hunger and fullness cues, mindful eaters are less likely to overeat and more likely to maintain a healthy weight.

- **Emotional Well-Being:** Mindful eating can help individuals develop a healthier relationship with food, reducing stress-related eating and emotional eating patterns.
- **Enhanced Enjoyment:** When you fully engage with your food, you're more likely to appreciate its flavors and textures, leading to a more satisfying eating experience.

Chapter 7: Portion Control Strategies

The Importance of Portion Control

Portion control plays a significant role in weight management by helping individuals regulate their calorie intake and prevent overeating. By becoming mindful of portion sizes, individuals can enjoy their favorite foods while still maintaining a healthy balance.

Mini Habits for Portion Control

Use Visual Cues: Familiarize yourself with common portion sizes by using visual aids such as measuring cups, food scales, or everyday objects (e.g., a deck of cards for protein portions).

Plate Method: Fill half your plate with non-starchy vegetables, one-quarter with lean protein, and one-quarter with whole grains or starchy vegetables.

Pre-Portion Snacks: Divide large snack packages into single-serving portions to prevent mindless overeating. Store pre-portioned snacks in grab-and-go containers for easy access.

Mindful Plating: Serve meals on smaller plates to create the illusion of larger portions. Avoid going back for seconds unless you're genuinely hungry.

Eat Slowly: Take your time to chew each bite thoroughly and savor the flavors. Eating slowly allows your body to register fullness more accurately, reducing the likelihood of overeating.

Practical Tips for Portion Control

Be Mindful of Restaurant Portions: Restaurant portions are often larger than necessary. Consider splitting a meal with a dining companion or asking for a to-go box to save half for later.

Practice the Two-Bite Rule: If you're indulging in a treat or dessert, limit yourself to two satisfying bites. This allows you to enjoy the flavor without overdoing it.

Pay Attention to Serving Sizes: Check food labels for recommended serving sizes and adjust your portions accordingly. Be mindful of hidden calories in condiments, dressings, and sauces.

Long-Term Benefits of Portion Control

- **Stable Weight Management:** By maintaining portion control habits, individuals can more effectively manage their weight and prevent fluctuations.
- **Healthy Eating Patterns:** Portion control encourages a balanced approach to eating, focusing on nutrient-dense foods in appropriate amounts.
- **Improved Relationship with Food:** Practicing portion control fosters a healthier mindset around food, reducing feelings of guilt or deprivation associated with overeating.

Chapter 8: Healthy Food Choices

Promoting Nutritious Eating Habits

Making informed food choices is essential for overall health and well-being. By incorporating mini habits that prioritize nutrient-rich foods, individuals can optimize their diet and support long-term health goals.

Mini Habits for Healthier Eating

Fill Half Your Plate with Produce: Aim to include a variety of colorful fruits and vegetables in your meals. These foods are rich in vitamins, minerals, and antioxidants that support optimal health.

Choose Whole Grains: Opt for whole grains such as brown rice, quinoa, oats, and whole wheat bread over refined grains. Whole grains provide fiber, which aids digestion and helps keep you feeling full.

Prioritize Lean Proteins: Incorporate lean protein sources such as poultry, fish, tofu, beans, and legumes into your meals. Protein is essential for muscle repair and maintenance and can help keep you feeling satisfied between meals.

Include Healthy Fats: Incorporate sources of healthy fats such as avocados, nuts, seeds, and olive oil into your diet. These fats provide essential fatty acids that support brain health and help keep you feeling full.

Limit Added Sugars: Minimize your intake of foods and beverages high in added sugars, such as soda, candy, baked goods, and sugary cereals. Instead, satisfy your sweet tooth with naturally sweet foods like fruit.

Building a Balanced Plate

- **Vegetables:** Fill half your plate with a colorful assortment of vegetables, including leafy greens, cruciferous vegetables, and colorful peppers.
- **Protein:** Include a palm-sized portion of lean protein, such as grilled chicken breast, salmon, tofu, or beans.
- **Whole Grains:** Add a serving of whole grains or starchy vegetables to provide energy and fiber, such as brown rice, quinoa, sweet potatoes, or whole grain pasta.

- **Healthy Fats:** Include a small serving of healthy fats, such as sliced avocado, nuts, seeds, or a drizzle of olive oil, to provide flavor and satiety.

Tips for Healthy Eating

- Meal Prep: Spend time planning and preparing meals in advance to ensure you have nutritious options available throughout the week.
- Read Labels: Take the time to read food labels and ingredient lists to make informed choices about the foods you consume.
- Listen to Your Body: Pay attention to your body's hunger and fullness cues, eating when you're hungry and stopping when you're satisfied.

Long-Term Benefits of Healthy Eating

- **Reduced Risk of Chronic Disease:** A diet rich in fruits, vegetables, whole grains, and lean proteins can help reduce the risk of chronic diseases such as heart disease, diabetes, and certain cancers.
- **Improved Energy and Vitality:** Nutrient-dense foods provide the essential vitamins and minerals your body needs to function optimally, leading to increased energy levels and overall vitality.
- **Enhanced Mood and Well-Being:** Eating a balanced diet can positively impact mood and mental health, reducing the risk of depression and anxiety.

Chapter 9: Hydration Habits

The Importance of Hydration

Staying hydrated is essential for overall health and can support weight loss. Water helps regulate body temperature, aids digestion, and helps you feel full, which can reduce overeating.

Mini Habits for Better Hydration

Drink Water Before Meals: Make it a habit to drink a glass of water before each meal. This can help you feel fuller and reduce the amount of food you eat.

- **Carry a Water Bottle:** Keep a reusable water bottle with you throughout the day. Having water readily available encourages regular drinking.
- **Set Reminders:** Use alarms or smartphone apps to remind you to drink water at regular intervals.
- **Flavor Your Water:** If you find plain water boring, add natural flavor with slices of lemon, lime, cucumber, or mint. This can make drinking water more enjoyable.
- **Track Your Intake:** Use a water tracking app or a journal to keep track of how much water you drink each day. Aim for at least 8 cups (64 ounces) of water daily, or more if you're active or in a hot climate.

Benefits of Staying Hydrated

- **Appetite Control:** Drinking water can help control hunger and prevent overeating. Sometimes, thirst is mistaken for hunger.
- **Increased Energy:** Proper hydration helps maintain energy levels and can reduce feelings of fatigue.
- **Improved Digestion:** Water aids digestion and helps prevent constipation.
- **Better Skin Health:** Staying hydrated supports healthy skin by keeping it moisturized and aiding in detoxification.

Chapter 10: Smart Snacking

The Role of Snacking in Weight Loss

Snacking can either support or sabotage your weight loss efforts. Healthy snacks can keep your energy levels stable and prevent overeating at meals, while unhealthy snacks can add unnecessary calories and hinder progress.

Mini Habits for Smart Snacking

- **Plan Your Snacks:** Plan and prepare healthy snacks in advance. Having nutritious options readily available can prevent impulsive, unhealthy choices.
- **Choose Whole Foods:** Opt for whole foods like fruits, vegetables, nuts, and yogurt. These snacks are nutrient-dense and satisfying.

- **Portion Control:** Pre-portion snacks into single-serving sizes. This helps prevent overeating and makes it easier to grab a healthy option on the go.
- **Include Protein and Fiber:** Choose snacks that contain protein and fiber, such as apple slices with peanut butter or a handful of nuts. Protein and fiber help keep you full longer.
- **Avoid Sugary Snacks:** Limit sugary snacks and beverages, which can cause energy spikes and crashes. Opt for naturally sweet options like fruit.

Healthy Snack Ideas

- **Fresh Fruit:** Apples, bananas, berries, and grapes are convenient and nutritious options.
- **Vegetables and Hummus:** Carrot sticks, cucumber slices, and bell pepper strips paired with hummus make a satisfying snack.
- **Nuts and Seeds:** A small handful of almonds, walnuts, or sunflower seeds provides healthy fats and protein.
- **Greek Yogurt:** Greek yogurt is high in protein and can be paired with fruit or a sprinkle of nuts.

Benefits of Smart Snacking

- **Stable Energy Levels:** Healthy snacks provide a steady source of energy throughout the day, preventing energy crashes and maintaining focus.
- **Weight Management:** Nutrient-dense snacks can help control hunger and prevent overeating at meals, supporting weight management goals.

- **Improved Nutrient Intake:** Smart snacking increases the intake of essential nutrients, contributing to overall health and well-being.

Chapter 11: Meal Planning and Preparation

The Importance of Meal Planning

Meal planning and preparation are powerful tools for maintaining a healthy diet. By planning your meals in advance, you can ensure you have nutritious options available, reduce the temptation to make unhealthy choices, and save time and money.

Mini Habits for Effective Meal Planning

- **Create a Weekly Menu:** Spend a few minutes each week planning your meals. Write down your meal plan and create a corresponding shopping list.
- **Prep Ingredients in Advance:** Chop vegetables, marinate proteins, and prepare grains in advance to make meal preparation quicker and easier during the week.
- **Batch Cooking:** Cook larger quantities of meals and store them in portioned containers for easy grab-and-go options. Batch cooking is especially useful for busy weekdays.
- **Use Leftovers Wisely:** Incorporate leftovers into new meals to minimize food waste and save time. For

example, use leftover roasted vegetables in a salad or wrap.
- **Stock Up on Essentials:** Keep your pantry stocked with healthy staples such as whole grains, beans, canned tomatoes, and spices to make meal preparation easier.

Benefits of Meal Planning and Preparation

- **Reduced Stress:** Knowing what you'll eat ahead of time eliminates the stress of last-minute meal decisions and helps you stick to your healthy eating goals.
- **Improved Nutrition:** Planning meals ensures a balanced intake of nutrients and prevents reliance on unhealthy convenience foods.
- **Cost Savings:** Meal planning allows you to buy only what you need, reducing food waste and saving money on groceries.

Chapter 12: Grocery Shopping Strategies

Smart Grocery Shopping

Making healthy food choices starts with smart grocery shopping. By adopting mini habits that focus on nutritious foods, you can set yourself up for success and make healthier eating easier.

Mini Habits for Smart Grocery Shopping

- **Shop the Perimeter:** Focus on the outer aisles of the grocery store where fresh produce, lean proteins, and dairy products are typically located. Avoid the inner aisles where processed and packaged foods are more common.
- **Read Labels:** Take the time to read food labels and ingredient lists. Look for products with minimal ingredients and avoid items high in added sugars, unhealthy fats, and sodium.
- **Stick to Your List:** Create a shopping list based on your meal plan and stick to it. This helps prevent impulse purchases and ensures you have the ingredients you need for healthy meals.
- **Buy in Bulk:** Purchase staples like grains, beans, nuts, and seeds in bulk to save money and reduce packaging waste. Store bulk items in airtight containers to maintain freshness.
- **Choose Seasonal Produce:** Opt for fruits and vegetables that are in season for better flavor and nutritional value. Seasonal produce is often more affordable and environmentally friendly.

Benefits of Smart Grocery Shopping

- **Healthier Food Choices:** By prioritizing fresh, whole foods, you can create a nutritious diet that supports overall health and well-being.
- **Reduced Food Waste:** Planning your grocery shopping and sticking to a list helps minimize food waste and ensures you use what you buy.

- **Cost Savings:** Buying in bulk and choosing seasonal produce can save money and make healthy eating more affordable.

Chapter 13: Overcoming Common Eating Challenges

Addressing Eating Challenges

Many individuals face common challenges when it comes to maintaining healthy eating habits. By adopting mini habits to address these challenges, you can stay on track and achieve your dietary goals.

Mini Habits for Overcoming Eating Challenges

- **Emotional Eating:** When you feel the urge to eat due to emotions, pause and assess your feelings. Engage in alternative activities such as going for a walk, practicing deep breathing, or talking to a friend.
- **Social Situations:** Plan ahead for social events by eating a healthy snack before you go, bringing a nutritious dish to share, and practicing mindful eating to avoid overeating.
- **Dining Out:** Make healthier choices when dining out by choosing grilled or baked options, requesting dressings and sauces on the side, and controlling portion sizes by sharing a meal or taking half home.

- **Cravings:** Manage cravings by keeping healthy snacks on hand, staying hydrated, and allowing yourself occasional treats in moderation to avoid feelings of deprivation.
- **Busy Schedules:** Plan and prepare meals in advance to ensure you have healthy options available even on busy days. Utilize slow cookers, instant pots, and batch cooking to save time.

Benefits of Addressing Eating Challenges

- **Improved Self-Control:** Developing strategies to overcome eating challenges enhances self-control and supports long-term healthy eating habits.
- **Reduced Stress:** By having a plan in place to address common challenges, you can reduce the stress and anxiety associated with maintaining a healthy diet.
- **Increased Success:** Overcoming eating challenges increases your likelihood of achieving and maintaining your dietary and weight management goals.

By incorporating these mini habits into your daily routine, you can develop a healthier relationship with food, make more nutritious choices, and support long-term weight management and overall well-being. Remember, small changes can lead to significant results over time.

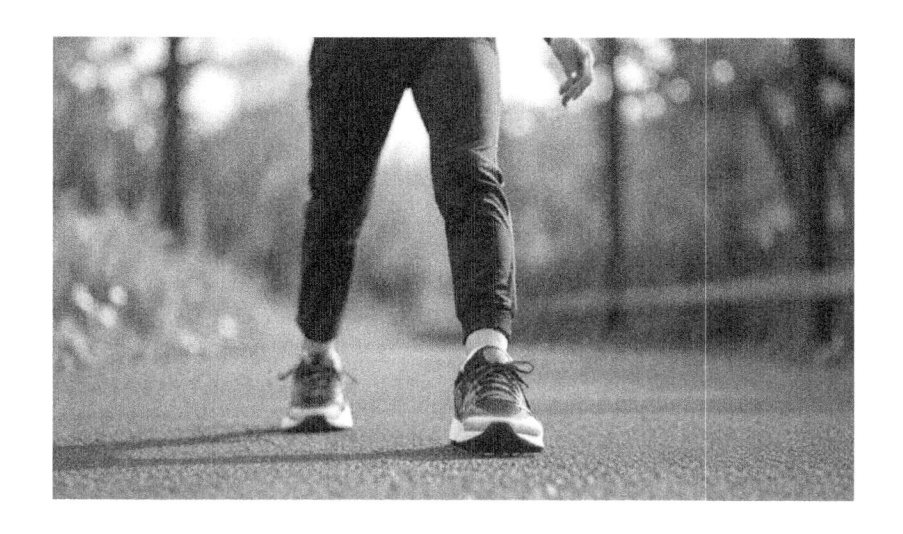

Part 3: Mini Habits for Exercise

"Weight loss doesn't begin in the gym with a dumbbell. It starts in your head with a decision."

Unknown

Chapter 14: The Power of Daily Movement

Understanding the Importance of Daily Movement

Regular physical activity is crucial for maintaining a healthy weight, improving cardiovascular health, and enhancing overall well-being. Integrating daily movement into your routine can have profound effects on both your physical and mental health.

Mini Habits for Increasing Daily Movement

Take the Stairs: Whenever possible, opt for stairs instead of elevators or escalators. This small habit can significantly increase your daily physical activity.

Walk More: Aim to walk for at least 10 minutes after meals or incorporate short walks into your daily routine. Use a pedometer or smartphone app to track your steps and set gradual goals to increase them.

Stand Up Frequently: If you have a sedentary job, set a timer to remind yourself to stand up and stretch every 30-60 minutes. Consider using a standing desk for part of the day.

Active Commutes: If feasible, walk or bike to work or school. If you use public transportation, get off one stop early and walk the rest of the way.

Household Chores: Engage in household chores like vacuuming, gardening, or washing the car. These activities not only keep your home tidy but also help you stay active.

Benefits of Daily Movement

- **Improved Cardiovascular Health:** Regular movement strengthens the heart and improves circulation, reducing the risk of cardiovascular diseases.
- **Increased Energy Levels:** Physical activity boosts energy by enhancing blood flow and oxygen supply to muscles and tissues.

- **Better Mood:** Exercise releases endorphins, which can improve mood and reduce stress and anxiety.
- **Weight Management:** Regular physical activity helps burn calories, contributing to weight loss and maintenance.

Chapter 15: Incorporating Strength Training

The Importance of Strength Training

Strength training is essential for building and maintaining muscle mass, improving bone density, and boosting metabolism. It complements cardiovascular exercise by providing a balanced approach to fitness.

Mini Habits for Strength Training

Bodyweight Exercises: Start with simple bodyweight exercises like squats, push-ups, lunges, and planks. These exercises can be done anywhere and don't require any equipment.

Short Workouts: Incorporate short, 5-10 minute strength training sessions into your day. Focus on different muscle groups each day for a balanced workout routine.

Resistance Bands: Use resistance bands for added resistance during your workouts. They are portable, affordable, and effective for strength training.

Strength Training Classes: Join a class or follow online videos that provide guided strength training workouts. This can help with motivation and ensure proper form.

Incremental Increases: Gradually increase the weight or resistance you use in your exercises. Small, consistent increases help build strength over time without causing injury.

Benefits of Strength Training

- **Increased Muscle Mass:** Strength training helps build and maintain muscle mass, which is crucial for overall strength and metabolic health.
- **Enhanced Metabolism:** Muscle tissue burns more calories at rest than fat tissue, helping to increase your resting metabolic rate.
- **Improved Bone Health:** Weight-bearing exercises improve bone density and reduce the risk of osteoporosis.
- **Functional Fitness:** Strength training improves functional fitness, making daily activities easier and reducing the risk of injury.

Chapter 16: Making Cardio Fun

The Role of Cardiovascular Exercise

Cardiovascular exercise is vital for heart health, endurance, and calorie burning. Finding enjoyable ways to incorporate cardio can make it easier to stick with a regular routine.

Mini Habits for Enjoyable Cardio

Dance: Turn on your favorite music and dance around your living room. Dancing is a fun way to get your heart rate up and burn calories.

Play Sports: Engage in sports or recreational activities you enjoy, such as basketball, soccer, tennis, or swimming. These activities provide a great cardio workout while being enjoyable.

Jump Rope: Keep a jump rope handy for quick cardio sessions. Jumping rope is an effective, high-intensity workout that can be done in short bursts.

Active Video Games: Play video games that require physical movement, such as those on the Wii, Kinect, or VR platforms. These games make exercise fun and interactive.

Join a Class: Participate in group fitness classes like Zumba, spinning, or aerobics. The social aspect and energetic atmosphere can make cardio workouts more enjoyable.

Benefits of Cardiovascular Exercise

- **Heart Health:** Regular cardio strengthens the heart and improves its efficiency, reducing the risk of heart disease.
- **Weight Loss:** Cardiovascular exercise burns calories, aiding in weight loss and weight maintenance.
- **Increased Endurance:** Cardio improves stamina and endurance, making daily activities easier and enhancing overall physical performance.

- **Mental Health:** Cardiovascular exercise releases endorphins, which help reduce stress, anxiety, and depression.

Chapter 17: Flexibility and Stretching
The Importance of Flexibility

Flexibility is a key component of overall fitness, contributing to improved range of motion, reduced injury risk, and enhanced physical performance. Regular stretching helps maintain flexibility and prevent muscle tightness.

Mini Habits for Flexibility

Morning Stretch: Start your day with a 5-minute stretching routine to wake up your muscles and increase blood flow.

Post-Workout Stretch: Always end your workout with a few minutes of stretching to cool down and improve flexibility.

Yoga or Pilates: Incorporate yoga or Pilates into your routine. These practices emphasize stretching and flexibility, and can be done in short sessions.

Desk Stretches: Perform simple stretches at your desk throughout the day to relieve tension and prevent stiffness from prolonged sitting.

Dynamic Stretching: Before workouts, engage in dynamic stretches like leg swings and arm circles to warm up your muscles and prepare them for activity.

Benefits of Flexibility and Stretching

- **Improved Range of Motion:** Stretching enhances flexibility and range of motion, making daily activities and physical exercises easier.
- **Injury Prevention:** Flexible muscles and joints are less prone to injuries. Stretching helps prevent muscle strains and joint sprains.
- **Reduced Muscle Tension:** Regular stretching relieves muscle tension and reduces the risk of muscle imbalances.
- **Enhanced Relaxation:** Stretching promotes relaxation and reduces stress, contributing to overall mental well-being.

Chapter 18: Building an Exercise Routine

Creating a Balanced Exercise Routine

A well-rounded exercise routine includes a mix of cardiovascular exercise, strength training, and flexibility work. Consistency and variety are key to maintaining an effective and enjoyable fitness program.

Mini Habits for Building a Routine

Start Small: Begin with short, manageable workout sessions. Gradually increase the duration and intensity as you build endurance and strength.

Schedule Workouts: Treat your workouts like appointments. Schedule them into your calendar and prioritize them to ensure consistency.

Mix It Up: Incorporate a variety of exercises to keep your routine interesting and work different muscle groups. This prevents boredom and improves overall fitness.

Track Your Progress: Keep a workout journal or use a fitness app to track your progress. Recording your workouts helps you stay motivated and see your improvements over time.

Set Realistic Goals: Set achievable fitness goals that are specific, measurable, and time-bound. Celebrate your successes and adjust your goals as you progress.

Benefits of a Balanced Routine

- **Comprehensive Fitness:** A balanced routine improves cardiovascular health, builds muscle, and enhances flexibility, leading to overall physical fitness.

- **Reduced Boredom:** Mixing different types of exercises keeps your routine interesting and prevents burnout.
- **Consistent Progress:** Tracking progress and setting goals helps maintain motivation and ensures continuous improvement.
- **Increased Motivation:** Seeing your progress and achieving milestones boosts motivation and commitment to your fitness journey.

Chapter 19: Overcoming Exercise Barriers

Addressing Common Exercise Barriers

Many people face barriers to regular exercise, such as lack of time, motivation, or resources. Identifying and overcoming these barriers is essential for maintaining a consistent fitness routine.

Mini Habits for Overcoming Barriers

Time Management: Break workouts into shorter sessions that fit into your schedule. Even 10-minute sessions throughout the day can add up.

Stay Motivated: Find a workout buddy, join a fitness group, or participate in online challenges to stay motivated and accountable.

Home Workouts: Utilize bodyweight exercises, resistance bands, or online workout videos to create effective home workouts without needing a gym membership.

Set a Routine: Establish a regular workout schedule that fits your lifestyle. Consistency helps make exercise a habit.

Find Enjoyable Activities: Choose physical activities you enjoy to make exercise more fun and sustainable. This could be dancing, hiking, playing sports, or participating in group fitness classes.

Benefits of Overcoming Exercise Barriers

- **Improved Consistency:** Addressing barriers helps establish a regular exercise routine, leading to long-term fitness and health benefits.
- **Increased Enjoyment:** Finding enjoyable activities makes exercise more appealing and less of a chore.
- **Enhanced Motivation:** Overcoming obstacles boosts confidence and motivation to continue with your fitness journey.
- **Better Health Outcomes:** Regular exercise contributes to improved physical and mental health, enhancing overall quality of life.

Chapter 20: Staying Active Throughout the Day

The Importance of Staying Active

In addition to scheduled workouts, staying active throughout the day is crucial for maintaining overall health. Sedentary behavior can negate the benefits of exercise, so it's important to incorporate movement into daily activities.

Mini Habits for Staying Active

Walk More: Take short walks throughout the day, especially after meals. Aim for at least 10,000 steps daily.

Active Breaks: Take active breaks during work or study sessions. Stretch, walk around, or do a few quick exercises to break up long periods of sitting.

Stand More: Use a standing desk or take phone calls standing up. Standing burns more calories than sitting and reduces the risk of sedentary-related health issues.

Household Activities: Engage in active household chores like cleaning, gardening, or DIY projects. These activities keep you moving and contribute to daily physical activity.

Play with Pets: If you have pets, spend time playing with them or taking them for walks. This not only keeps you active but also strengthens your bond with your pets.

Benefits of Staying Active

- **Improved Circulation:** Regular movement improves blood flow and reduces the risk of circulatory problems.

- **Reduced Sedentary Time:** Staying active throughout the day reduces the negative health impacts associated with prolonged sitting.
- **Increased Calorie Burn:** Daily activities and active breaks contribute to overall calorie expenditure, supporting weight management.
- **Enhanced Well-Being:** Staying active boosts energy levels, mood, and overall well-being.

By incorporating these mini habits for exercise into your daily routine, you can create a sustainable and effective fitness program that supports your weight loss goals and overall health. Remember, consistency and enjoyment are key to long-term success. Small, manageable changes can lead to significant improvements in your physical and mental well-being.

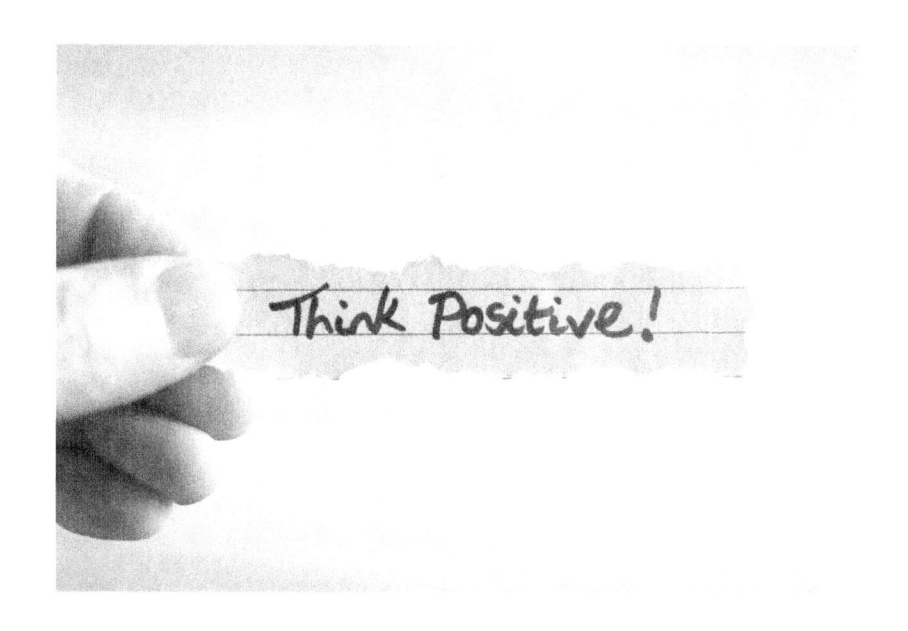

Part 4: Mindset and Motivation

"If you don't take time to take care of your health now, you're gonna have to make time for feeling sick and tired later."

Chapter 21: Understanding the Power of Mindset

The Role of Mindset in Weight Loss

Mindset plays a crucial role in achieving and maintaining weight loss. A positive and growth-oriented mindset can help you overcome obstacles, stay motivated, and make healthier choices consistently. Understanding and cultivating the right mindset is essential for long-term success.

Types of Mindsets

Fixed Mindset: Believing that your abilities and traits are fixed and cannot be changed. This mindset can lead to giving up easily when faced with challenges.

Growth Mindset: Believing that you can develop your abilities through effort, learning, and persistence. This mindset encourages resilience and continuous improvement.

Mini Habits for Developing a Growth Mindset

Practice Self-Compassion: Treat yourself with kindness and understanding, especially when you encounter setbacks. Recognize that everyone makes mistakes and that these are opportunities for growth.

Set Learning Goals: Focus on learning and personal development rather than just outcome-based goals. For example, aim to learn more about nutrition and exercise rather than just aiming for a specific weight.

Embrace Challenges: View challenges as opportunities to grow and improve. Instead of avoiding difficult situations, face them with a problem-solving attitude.

Celebrate Effort: Acknowledge and celebrate the effort you put into making healthy choices, regardless of the immediate outcome. This reinforces positive behavior and builds confidence.

Positive Affirmations: Use positive affirmations to reinforce a growth mindset. Statements like "I am capable of change" and "Every step forward is progress" can help shift your perspective.

Benefits of a Growth Mindset

- **Increased Resilience:** A growth mindset helps you bounce back from setbacks and continue working towards your goals.
- **Enhanced Motivation:** Focusing on learning and improvement keeps you motivated even when progress is slow.
- **Improved Self-Efficacy:** Believing in your ability to change and grow boosts your confidence and willingness to take on new challenges.
- Long-Term Success: A growth mindset supports sustainable habits and continuous personal development, leading to lasting weight loss and overall well-being.

Chapter 22: Setting SMART Goals

The Importance of Goal Setting

Setting clear and achievable goals is essential for staying focused and motivated on your weight loss journey. SMART goals—Specific, Measurable, Achievable, Relevant, and Time-bound—provide a structured approach to goal setting.

Mini Habits for Setting SMART Goals

Specific: Define your goals clearly and precisely. Instead of saying "I want to lose weight," specify "I want to lose 10 pounds in three months."

Measurable: Ensure your goals are measurable so you can track your progress. For example, "I will walk for 30 minutes, five days a week" allows you to monitor your activity.

Achievable: Set realistic and attainable goals. Aim for small, incremental changes that are within your reach.

Relevant: Align your goals with your overall objectives and values. Ensure that your goals are meaningful and contribute to your long-term vision of health and well-being.

Time-bound: Set a deadline for achieving your goals. This creates a sense of urgency and helps you stay focused. For example, "I will reduce my sugar intake by half within the next month."

Benefits of SMART Goals

- **Clarity and Focus:** SMART goals provide clear direction and help you stay focused on what matters.
- **Motivation:** Achievable and relevant goals keep you motivated and committed to your weight loss journey.
- **Accountability:** Measurable and time-bound goals enable you to track your progress and hold yourself accountable.

- **Sense of Achievement:** Achieving specific, incremental goals boosts your confidence and encourages further progress.

Chapter 23: Building a Support System

The Role of Social Support

A strong support system is vital for staying motivated and overcoming challenges. Friends, family, and communities can provide encouragement, accountability, and practical help on your weight loss journey.

Mini Habits for Building a Support System

Communicate Your Goals: Share your weight loss goals with supportive friends and family members. This helps create a network of people who understand and support your efforts.

Find a Workout Buddy: Partner with a friend or family member for workouts. Exercising with someone else can make it more enjoyable and provide mutual motivation.

Join a Group: Participate in weight loss or fitness groups, either in person or online. These groups can offer encouragement, share tips, and provide a sense of community.

Seek Professional Help: Consider working with a nutritionist, personal trainer, or therapist. Professional guidance can provide personalized support and expert advice.

Celebrate Together: Share your successes and milestones with your support system. Celebrating achievements with others reinforces positive behavior and strengthens your motivation.

Benefits of a Support System

- **Increased Motivation:** Supportive relationships provide encouragement and help you stay motivated.
- **Accountability:** Sharing your goals and progress with others creates accountability and reduces the likelihood of giving up.
- **Emotional Support:** Friends and family can offer emotional support during difficult times, helping you navigate challenges more effectively.
- **Shared Knowledge:** Support systems can provide valuable insights, tips, and resources to help you achieve your goals.

Chapter 24: Overcoming Plateaus

Understanding Weight Loss Plateaus

Weight loss plateaus are common and can be frustrating. They occur when your body adapts to your current routine, leading to a slowdown or halt in weight loss progress. Understanding and overcoming plateaus is crucial for continued success.

Mini Habits for Overcoming Plateaus

Reassess Your Goals: Review your goals and make necessary adjustments. Ensure they are still challenging and relevant to your current situation.

Mix Up Your Routine: Introduce variety into your exercise and diet. Try new workouts, increase intensity, or experiment with different healthy foods.

Monitor Your Intake: Track your food intake more closely. Small changes in portion sizes or food choices can add up over time and impact your progress.

Stay Hydrated: Ensure you are drinking enough water. Proper hydration is essential for metabolism and overall health.

Prioritize Sleep: Make sure you are getting enough quality sleep. Lack of sleep can negatively affect metabolism and weight loss.

Benefits of Overcoming Plateaus

- **Renewed Progress:** Breaking through a plateau allows you to continue making progress towards your weight loss goals.
- **Increased Motivation:** Successfully overcoming a plateau boosts your confidence and motivation to keep going.
- **Improved Adaptability:** Learning to adapt your routine helps you become more flexible and resilient in the face of challenges.

- **Better Understanding:** Analyzing and adjusting your approach provides valuable insights into your body's responses to diet and exercise.

Chapter 25: Dealing with Setbacks

Accepting and Learning from Setbacks

Setbacks are a natural part of any weight loss journey. Instead of viewing them as failures, see them as opportunities to learn and grow. Developing strategies to deal with setbacks is essential for long-term success.

Mini Habits for Dealing with Setbacks

Reflect and Learn: Take time to reflect on what led to the setback. Identify any patterns or triggers and think about how you can address them in the future.

Practice Self-Compassion: Be kind to yourself and avoid negative self-talk. Understand that setbacks are part of the process and do not define your overall progress.

Reframe Your Mindset: View setbacks as temporary and solvable. Use them as motivation to refocus and recommit to your goals.

Create a Plan: Develop a specific plan to get back on track. This could include adjusting your diet, recommitting to your exercise routine, or seeking additional support.

Celebrate Small Wins: Focus on the positive aspects and small victories, even during setbacks. Recognize your efforts and progress to maintain a positive outlook.

Benefits of Dealing with Setbacks

- **Resilience:** Learning to handle setbacks builds resilience and strengthens your ability to cope with future challenges.
- **Increased Motivation:** Successfully overcoming setbacks can reignite your motivation and commitment to your goals.
- **Improved Problem-Solving:** Addressing setbacks enhances your problem-solving skills and helps you develop more effective strategies.
- **Positive Mindset:** Embracing setbacks as part of the journey fosters a positive and growth-oriented mindset.

Chapter 26: Cultivating Patience and Persistence

The Importance of Patience and Persistence

Weight loss is a gradual process that requires patience and persistence. Cultivating these qualities helps you stay committed and focused, even when progress is slow or challenges arise.

Mini Habits for Cultivating Patience and Persistence

Set Realistic Expectations: Understand that significant weight loss takes time. Set realistic and achievable goals to maintain motivation and avoid frustration.

Focus on Progress, Not Perfection: Celebrate incremental progress and small victories. Avoid striving for perfection, as it can lead to disappointment and burnout.

Maintain Consistency: Stick to your healthy habits and routines, even when results are not immediate. Consistency is key to long-term success.

Stay Positive: Keep a positive attitude and remind yourself of your long-term goals. Positive thinking can help you stay motivated and persistent.

Seek Support: Lean on your support system for encouragement and motivation. Sharing your journey with others can help you stay accountable and focused.

Benefits of Patience and Persistence

- **Sustainable Weight Loss:** Patience and persistence promote sustainable weight loss and healthy habits that can be maintained over the long term.
- **Reduced Stress:** Accepting that weight loss is a gradual process reduces stress and anxiety, allowing you to enjoy the journey.
- **Improved Mental Health:** A positive and patient mindset enhances mental well-being and reduces the risk of negative self-talk and discouragement.

- **Long-Term Success:** Persistence ensures that you stay committed to your goals, leading to lasting success and improved health.

Chapter 27: Creating a Positive Environment

The Influence of Environment on Weight Loss

Your environment significantly impacts your ability to stick to healthy habits and achieve your weight loss goals. Creating a positive and supportive environment can make it easier to make healthy choices consistently.

Mini Habits for Creating a Positive Environment

Organize Your Kitchen: Keep healthy foods visible and easily accessible. Store unhealthy snacks out of sight to reduce temptation.

Plan Your Meals: Prepare healthy meals and snacks in advance to ensure you have nutritious options readily available.

Create a Workout Space: Designate a space in your home for exercise. Having a dedicated area for physical activity can make it easier to stick to your workout routine.

Surround Yourself with Support: Spend time with people who support your weight loss goals. Positive influences can help you stay motivated and committed.

Limit Negative Influences: Reduce exposure to negative influences that may hinder your progress, such as unhealthy food advertisements or unsupportive individuals.

Benefits of a Positive Environment

- **Reduced Temptation:** An environment that supports healthy choices reduces the likelihood of giving in to unhealthy temptations.
- **Increased Motivation:** A positive environment provides motivation and encouragement, making it easier to stay committed to your goals.
- **Improved Consistency:** Having healthy options readily available and a designated workout space promotes consistency in your habits.
- **Enhanced Well-Being:** A supportive environment contributes to overall well-being and reduces stress, making it easier to focus on your weight loss journey.

Chapter 28: Practicing Mindfulness and Stress Management

The Role of Mindfulness in Weight Loss

Mindfulness involves paying attention to the present moment without judgment. Practicing mindfulness can help you become more aware of your eating habits, reduce stress, and improve your overall relationship with food.

Mini Habits for Practicing Mindfulness

Mindful Eating: Pay attention to your food while eating. Savor each bite, chew slowly, and focus on the flavors and textures.

Body Scans: Practice body scans to become more aware of your physical sensations. This can help you identify hunger and fullness cues more accurately.

Breathing Exercises: Incorporate deep breathing exercises into your daily routine. Deep breathing helps reduce stress and promote relaxation.

Meditation: Spend a few minutes each day meditating. Meditation can improve mindfulness, reduce stress, and enhance overall well-being.

Gratitude Journaling: Keep a gratitude journal to focus on positive aspects of your life. This practice can boost your mood and help you stay motivated.

Benefits of Mindfulness and Stress Management

Improved Eating Habits: Mindfulness helps you become more aware of your eating habits, leading to healthier choices and better portion control.

Reduced Stress: Stress management techniques reduce stress levels, which can prevent stress-related eating and improve overall well-being.

Enhanced Awareness: Mindfulness increases awareness of your body's signals, helping you recognize hunger and fullness cues more accurately.

Better Mental Health: Mindfulness and stress management improve mental health, reducing the risk of anxiety and depression.

Chapter 29: Building Self-Discipline

The Importance of Self-Discipline

Self-discipline is essential for sticking to your weight loss plan and making healthy choices consistently. Developing self-discipline helps you resist temptations and stay focused on your goals.

Mini Habits for Building Self-Discipline

Start Small: Begin with small, manageable tasks to build your self-discipline gradually. For example, commit to a short daily walk or a single healthy meal each day.

Create a Routine: Establish a daily routine that includes healthy habits. Consistency in your routine strengthens self-discipline over time.

Set Clear Boundaries: Define clear boundaries for your eating and exercise habits. For example, limit junk food to specific occasions or set a regular workout schedule.

Use Reminders: Use reminders and cues to reinforce your healthy habits. Set alarms, post notes, or use apps to keep you on track.

Practice Delayed Gratification: Train yourself to delay gratification by setting small rewards for achieving specific milestones. This practice strengthens your ability to resist immediate temptations.

Benefits of Self-Discipline

- **Consistent Progress:** Self-discipline helps you maintain consistent progress towards your weight loss goals.
- **Improved Decision-Making:** Strong self-discipline improves your ability to make healthier choices, even in challenging situations.
- **Enhanced Self-Control: Developing** self-discipline increases your self-control, reducing the likelihood of impulsive eating or skipping workouts.
- **Long-Term Success: Self**-discipline supports sustainable habits and long-term weight loss success.

Chapter 30: Embracing the Journey

The Importance of Enjoying the Process

Weight loss is a journey that involves ups and downs. Embracing and enjoying the process can help you stay motivated and committed, making it easier to achieve your goals.

Mini Habits for Embracing the Journey

Focus on Non-Scale Victories: Celebrate non-scale victories such as increased energy, improved fitness, or better mood. These successes are important markers of progress.

Practice Gratitude: Regularly reflect on and express gratitude for your health, body, and the progress you've made. Gratitude helps maintain a positive outlook.

Be Patient: Understand that weight loss is a gradual process. Practice patience and avoid rushing the journey.

Find Joy in Healthy Habits: Discover activities and foods you enjoy that contribute to your weight loss goals. This makes the journey more enjoyable and sustainable.

Reflect on Your Why: Regularly remind yourself of the reasons why you started your weight loss journey. Keeping your motivation in mind helps you stay focused and committed.

Benefits of Embracing the Journey

- **Increased Motivation:** Enjoying the process keeps you motivated and engaged in your weight loss journey.
- **Improved Mental Health:** Focusing on positive aspects and practicing gratitude enhances mental well-being and reduces stress.
- **Sustainable Habits:** Finding joy in healthy habits makes them more sustainable and easier to maintain long-term.

- **Overall Well-Being:** Embracing the journey promotes overall well-being, making weight loss a positive and fulfilling experience.

By focusing on mindset and motivation, you can create a strong foundation for your weight loss journey. Cultivating a positive mindset, setting SMART goals, building a support system, overcoming plateaus, dealing with setbacks, and practicing mindfulness and self-discipline are all essential components of long-term success. Embrace the journey, stay patient, and enjoy the process, knowing that every small step forward brings you closer to your goals and a healthier, happier life.

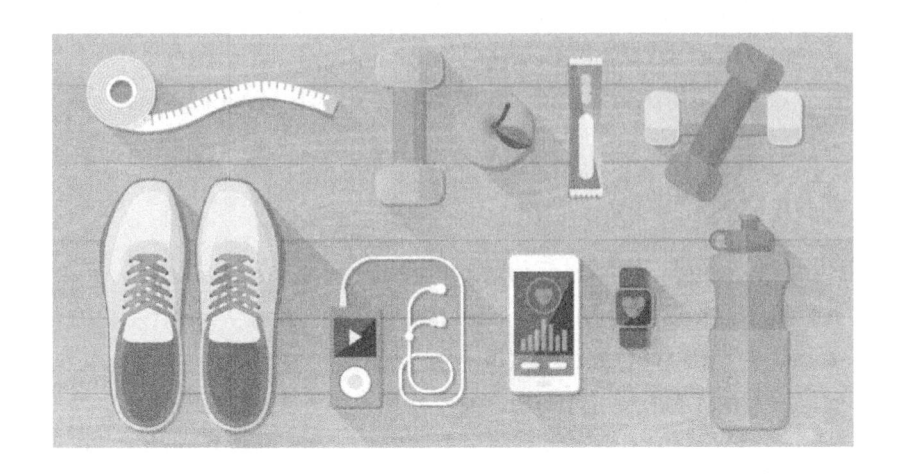

Conclusion: The Journey to Lasting Weight Loss

"The body achieves what the mind believes."

Reflecting on the Journey

As we conclude our exploration of mini habits for weight loss, it's essential to reflect on the journey you have undertaken. Weight loss is not merely about shedding pounds; it's about transforming your lifestyle, adopting healthier habits, and enhancing your overall well-being. This book has provided you with a comprehensive guide to making small, sustainable changes that can lead to significant, lasting results. Let's revisit the key concepts, reinforce their importance, and explore how to maintain your progress moving forward.

Revisiting the Mini Habits Approach

Mini habits are small, manageable actions that you can incorporate into your daily routine. These actions are so small that they seem almost trivial, but their cumulative effect can lead to substantial changes over time. The beauty of mini habits lies in their simplicity and the fact that they are easy to start and maintain. By focusing on small, consistent actions, you can build a foundation for long-term success without feeling overwhelmed.

Key Components of Mini Habits for Weight Loss

Nutrition:

Mindful Eating: Paying attention to what and how you eat helps you make healthier choices and enjoy your food more.

Portion Control: Managing portion sizes prevents overeating and helps you maintain a balanced diet.

Healthy Choices: Incorporating more fruits, vegetables, whole grains, and lean proteins into your diet supports weight loss and overall health.

Exercise:

Regular Physical Activity: Incorporating movement into your daily routine, whether through structured workouts or daily activities, boosts your metabolism and aids weight loss.

Strength Training: Building muscle mass through strength training exercises increases your resting metabolic rate and enhances your body composition.

Flexibility and Balance: Practices like yoga and stretching improve your flexibility, balance, and overall physical health.

Mindset and Motivation:

Growth Mindset: Believing in your ability to change and grow fosters resilience and continuous improvement.

SMART Goals: Setting Specific, Measurable, Achievable, Relevant, and Time-bound goals provides clear direction and accountability.

Support System: Building a network of supportive friends, family, and professionals helps you stay motivated and overcome challenges.

Behavioral Strategies:

Habit Formation: Consistently practicing mini habits leads to the formation of new, healthy habits that become automatic over time.

Overcoming Plateaus: Adjusting your routine and staying flexible helps you break through weight loss plateaus.

Dealing with Setbacks: Viewing setbacks as learning opportunities and practicing self-compassion ensures you stay on track.

Lifestyle Changes:

Sleep and Stress Management: Prioritizing quality sleep and managing stress through mindfulness and relaxation techniques supports overall health and weight loss.

Creating a Positive Environment: Organizing your physical and social environment to support your goals makes it easier to maintain healthy habits.

Sustainable Practices: Focusing on long-term, sustainable changes rather than quick fixes ensures lasting success.

The Importance of Consistency

Consistency is the cornerstone of any successful weight loss journey. While motivation can fluctuate, building consistent habits ensures that you continue to make progress even when motivation wanes. The mini habits approach emphasizes small, manageable actions that you can sustain over the long term. By committing to these small changes and practicing them consistently, you create a solid foundation for lasting weight loss and improved health.

Overcoming Common Challenges

Throughout your weight loss journey, you may encounter various challenges. Understanding these challenges and developing strategies to overcome them is crucial for long-term success.

Lack of Motivation: It's natural for motivation to ebb and flow. On days when you feel less motivated, rely on the habits you've built and remind yourself of your long-term goals. Setting smaller, immediate goals can also help rekindle your motivation.

Time Constraints: Many people struggle to find time for healthy habits. Prioritize your health by scheduling time for exercise and meal preparation, and look for opportunities to incorporate movement into your daily routine.

Emotional Eating: Emotional eating can derail your progress. Develop alternative coping strategies for stress, such as mindfulness, deep breathing, or engaging in a hobby. Keeping a food diary can also help you identify emotional eating patterns and address them.

Social Pressures: Social events and peer pressure can make it challenging to stick to your goals. Communicate your goals to your friends and family, and seek their support. Plan ahead for social events by choosing healthier options and practicing moderation.

Plateaus: Weight loss plateaus are common. To overcome them, reassess your routine, introduce variety into your diet and exercise regimen, and consider consulting a professional for personalized advice.

Maintaining Your Progress

Maintaining your weight loss and healthy habits is an ongoing process. Here are some strategies to help you stay on track:

Regular Check-Ins: Periodically review your goals and progress. Adjust your goals as needed to ensure they remain challenging and relevant.

Continuous Learning: Stay informed about nutrition, fitness, and health. Continuously learning helps you stay motivated and adapt to new information.

Flexibility: Be flexible with your approach. Life circumstances change, and being able to adapt your routine ensures long-term sustainability.

Celebrate Milestones: Acknowledge and celebrate your achievements, no matter how small. Celebrating milestones reinforces positive behavior and keeps you motivated.

Self-Compassion: Practice self-compassion and avoid negative self-talk. Treat yourself with kindness and understanding, especially during setbacks.

The Bigger Picture: Holistic Health

Weight loss is just one aspect of a broader picture of holistic health. A holistic approach considers not only physical health but also mental, emotional, and social well-being. By focusing on all aspects of your health, you create a balanced and fulfilling lifestyle.

Physical Health: Regular exercise, balanced nutrition, adequate sleep, and regular medical check-ups are essential components of physical health.

Mental Health: Managing stress, practicing mindfulness, and seeking professional help when needed supports mental health.

Emotional Health: Building strong emotional resilience, practicing self-care, and maintaining healthy relationships contribute to emotional well-being.

Social Health: Cultivating supportive relationships, engaging in social activities, and contributing to your community enhances social health.

Your Journey Ahead

As you move forward, remember that your weight loss journey is unique to you. There is no one-size-fits-all approach, and what works for someone else may not work for you. Embrace your individuality and tailor your habits and routines to suit your preferences and lifestyle.

Key Takeaways:

Mini Habits Matter: Small, consistent actions can lead to significant, lasting changes. Focus on building and maintaining mini habits that support your weight loss goals.

Mindset is Crucial: Cultivating a positive, growth-oriented mindset helps you stay resilient and motivated, even during challenges.

Support Systems are Vital: Surround yourself with supportive individuals who encourage and motivate you. Seek professional help when needed.

Consistency Over Perfection: Strive for consistency in your habits rather than perfection. Small, consistent efforts yield better results than sporadic, intense efforts.

Holistic Health: Consider all aspects of your health—physical, mental, emotional, and social. A balanced approach ensures overall well-being.

Final Thoughts

Embarking on a weight loss journey is a commendable decision that requires dedication, effort, and perseverance. By incorporating mini habits into your daily routine, you have the tools to achieve sustainable weight loss and improved health. Remember that every step you take, no matter how small, brings you closer to your goals.

Stay patient, stay persistent, and embrace the journey. Celebrate your progress, learn from your setbacks, and continue to grow. Your journey to lasting weight loss is a continuous process of self-improvement and self-discovery. You have the power to transform your life, one mini habit at a time.

Thank you for allowing this book to be part of your journey. Here's to your health, happiness, and lasting success.

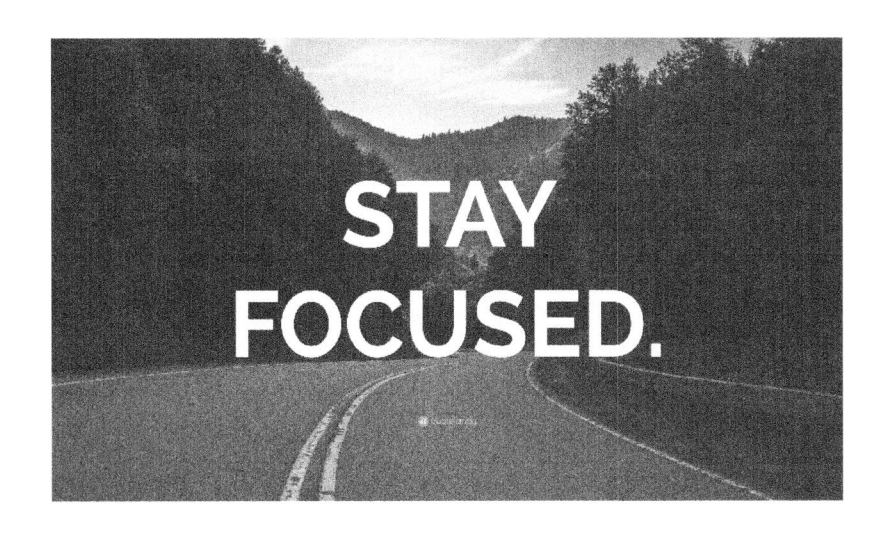

10 Motivational Quotes for Weight Loss

1. One day at a time.

2. The body achieves what the mind believes.

3. If you're going to doubt something, doubt your limits.

4. A goal without a plan is just a wish.

5. If you feel like quitting, think about why you started.

6. I can't change yesterday, but I can change today.

7. Your strongest muscle and your worst enemy is your mind, train it well.

8. Weight loss is not impossible. Weight loss is hard, but hard is not the same as impossible.

9. Motivation is what gets you started. Habit is what keeps you going.

10. Sacrifice is giving up something good for something better.

Offering Our Books

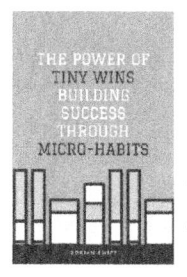

The Power of Tiny Wins Building Success Through Micro-Habits: Book about Tiny Habits for Tiny Wins - https://www.amazon.com/dp/B0CYFZNW35

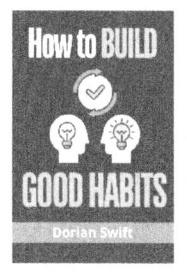

How to build good habits: Building Good Habits for Lasting Change https://www.amazon.com/dp/B0D5B5D5F3

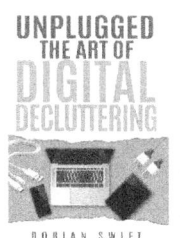

Unplugged: The Art of Digital Decluttering: How to Declutter Your Digital Life - https://www.amazon.com/dp/B0D4FHFMSG

Printed in Great Britain
by Amazon